Somatic Therapy Techniques for Beginners

The Self-Soothing Handbook for Trauma Release, Mind-Body Balance, and Resilience Building

Liz Press

Introduction

Welcome to "Somatic Therapy Techniques for Beginners: The Proven Self-Soothing Handbook for Trauma Release, Mind-Body Balance, and Resilience Building." In the journey of life, we encounter moments that shape us—some joyful, others challenging. For those navigating trauma, stress, or seeking to deepen their mind-body connection, this book serves as a guiding light.

Somatic therapy offers a unique approach, focusing on the intimate connection between our physical sensations, emotions, and mental well-being. Whether you're new to somatic practices or seeking to enrich your existing toolkit, this handbook empowers you with practical techniques designed to soothe your nervous system, foster resilience, and cultivate profound healing.

In these pages, we'll explore foundational techniques like grounding exercises, breathing practices, and progressive muscle relaxation—all tailored to help you reclaim a sense of safety and empowerment in your body. You'll discover how movement, touch, and mindfulness can serve as powerful allies in your journey toward healing. Beyond techniques, this book delves into understanding trauma responses, developing emotional resilience, and building a supportive framework for daily practice. Each chapter is crafted to provide clear, actionable steps that resonate with beginners and seasoned practitioners alike, ensuring accessibility without compromising depth.

Through real-life examples, case studies, and testimonials, you'll witness firsthand the transformative impact of somatic therapy on individuals' lives. Whether you're navigating past traumas, managing stress, or simply seeking greater balance, these insights will inspire and guide you toward sustainable well-being. As you embark on this journey, remember—you hold within you the innate capacity for healing. This book is your companion, offering tools to unlock that potential and embark on a path of self-discovery and growth. Together, let's embrace the wisdom of somatic therapy and embark on a journey toward resilience, balance, and a more vibrant life.

Chapter One

Understanding Somatic Therapy

What is Somatic Therapy?

Somatic therapy is an integrative approach to healing that emphasizes the connection between the mind and body. It is grounded in the belief that the body holds onto past traumas and that these physical manifestations can impact emotional and mental well-being. Unlike traditional talk therapies that focus predominantly on cognitive and emotional processes, somatic therapy addresses the physical sensations and bodily experiences that accompany psychological issues.

The term "somatic" comes from the Greek word "soma," which means "body." This form of therapy operates on the premise that the body and mind are intricately connected, and that emotional and psychological traumas can be stored within the body's tissues, muscles, and nervous system. Somatic therapy seeks to release these stored traumas and restore a sense of balance and harmony within the individual.

Practitioners of somatic therapy utilize a range of techniques to help clients become more aware of their bodily sensations and to release tension and trauma. These techniques may include breathing exercises, grounding practices, movement, touch, and body awareness exercises. By focusing on the body and its sensations, clients can access and process emotions and memories that might not be readily accessible through verbal communication alone. Somatic therapy is particularly effective for individuals who have experienced trauma, as traumatic experiences are often stored in the body and can manifest as physical symptoms such as chronic pain, tension, or fatigue. By addressing these physical manifestations, somatic therapy can help individuals process and heal from their traumatic experiences, leading to improved emotional and mental health.

The Science Behind Somatic Therapy

The science behind somatic therapy is rooted in an understanding of how the nervous system and the brain interact with the body. The autonomic nervous system (ANS), which regulates involuntary bodily functions such as heart rate, digestion, and respiratory rate, plays a crucial role in how the body responds to stress and trauma. The ANS is divided into two branches: the sympathetic nervous system (SNS) and the parasympathetic nervous system (PNS).

The sympathetic nervous system is responsible for the "fight or flight" response, which prepares the body to respond to perceived threats. When the SNS is activated, the body undergoes several physiological changes, such as increased heart rate, heightened alertness, and a release of stress hormones like adrenaline and cortisol. This response is crucial for survival, but when activated too frequently or intensely, it can lead to chronic stress and health problems.

The parasympathetic nervous system, on the other hand, is responsible for the "rest and digest" response, which helps the body relax and recover after a stressful event. When the PNS is activated, the body undergoes physiological changes that promote relaxation, such as decreased heart rate, slower breathing, and a reduction in stress hormone levels. A healthy balance between the SNS and PNS is essential for overall well-being.

Traumatic experiences can disrupt this balance by causing the nervous system to become stuck in a state of heightened arousal or shutdown. This can lead to a range of physical and psychological symptoms, such as anxiety, depression, chronic pain, and dissociation. Somatic therapy aims to restore balance to the nervous system by helping clients regulate their physiological responses to stress and trauma. One of the key mechanisms behind somatic therapy is the concept of neuroplasticity, which refers to the brain's ability to reorganize and adapt in response to new experiences. Through somatic practices, individuals can create new neural pathways that promote healing and resilience. By engaging in practices that promote body awareness and regulation, clients can retrain their nervous systems to respond more adaptively to stress and trauma.

Research has shown that somatic interventions can have a profound impact on the brain and body. For example, studies have demonstrated that practices such as deep breathing and mindfulness meditation can reduce the activity of the SNS and increase the activity of the PNS, leading to improved stress management and emotional regulation. Additionally, movement-based therapies, such as yoga and dance, have been shown to increase the release of endorphins and other feel-good neurotransmitters, promoting a sense of well-being and relaxation.

Benefits of Somatic Therapy

The benefits of somatic therapy are vast and multifaceted, encompassing physical, emotional, and psychological well-being. By addressing the body as an integral part of the healing process, somatic therapy offers a holistic approach that can lead to profound and lasting change. One of the primary benefits of somatic therapy is its ability to help individuals release stored trauma and tension from the body. Traumatic experiences can become "trapped" in the body's tissues, leading to chronic pain, tension, and other physical symptoms. Through somatic techniques, individuals can release these stored traumas, leading to relief from physical discomfort and an overall sense of relaxation and ease.

In addition to physical benefits, somatic therapy can also have a significant impact on emotional and psychological well-being. By fostering a greater sense of body awareness, individuals can become more attuned to their emotions and learn to recognize and process them in a healthy way. This increased emotional awareness can lead to improved emotional regulation and a greater sense of inner peace. Somatic therapy is particularly effective for individuals who have experienced trauma, as it provides a safe and supportive environment for processing traumatic memories and emotions. Traditional talk therapies can sometimes be re-traumatizing for individuals with a history of trauma, as they may be forced to relive painful memories through verbal recounting. Somatic therapy, on the other hand, allows individuals to process trauma in a non-verbal way, through the body. This can be a gentler and more effective approach for trauma survivors.

Another benefit of somatic therapy is its ability to improve the mind-body connection. In today's fast-paced and often stressful world, many individuals become disconnected from their bodies, leading to a range of physical and psychological issues. Somatic therapy helps individuals reconnect with their bodies, fostering a greater sense of embodiment and presence. This can lead to improved self-awareness, self-compassion, and overall well-being. Furthermore, somatic therapy can enhance resilience and coping skills. By learning to regulate their physiological responses to stress and trauma, individuals can become more resilient in the face of life's challenges. Somatic practices can help individuals build a "toolbox" of techniques for managing stress and emotions, promoting a greater sense of empowerment and self-efficacy.

How Somatic Therapy Differs from Other Modalities

Somatic therapy differs from other therapeutic modalities in several key ways, primarily in its focus on the body and its integration with the mind. While traditional talk therapies, such as cognitive-behavioral therapy (CBT) and psychodynamic therapy, focus on cognitive and emotional processes, somatic therapy emphasizes the importance of the body's role in healing. One of the main distinctions between somatic therapy and other modalities is its emphasis on body awareness and bodily sensations. In somatic therapy, clients are encouraged to tune into their bodies and notice physical sensations, such as tension, pain, or relaxation. This focus on the body allows individuals to access and process emotions and memories that may not be readily accessible through verbal communication alone.

Another key difference is the use of physical techniques in somatic therapy. While traditional talk therapies primarily involve verbal communication, somatic therapy incorporates a range of physical practices, such as breathing exercises, movement, touch, and grounding techniques. These practices help individuals release stored trauma and tension from the body, promoting physical and emotional healing. Somatic therapy also differs from other modalities in its approach to trauma. Traditional talk therapies can sometimes be re-traumatizing for individuals with a history of trauma, as they may be forced to relive painful memories through verbal recounting. Somatic therapy, on the other hand, provides a non-verbal way to process trauma, through the body. This can be a gentler and more effective approach for trauma survivors.

Furthermore, somatic therapy is holistic in nature, addressing the interconnectedness of the mind, body, and emotions. This holistic approach recognizes that physical, emotional, and psychological well-being are interrelated and that healing must involve all aspects of the self. By addressing the body as an integral part of the healing process, somatic therapy offers a comprehensive and integrated approach to well-being.

Chapter Two

The Mind-Body Connection

Understanding the Mind-Body Relationship

The mind-body relationship is a fundamental aspect of human existence, encompassing the intricate interplay between our mental and physical states. This connection is rooted in the understanding that our thoughts, emotions, and behaviors are closely linked to our physiological processes. Historically, the mind and body were often viewed as separate entities, but modern science has increasingly recognized their profound interconnectedness. This holistic perspective acknowledges that our mental state can significantly impact our physical health, and vice versa.

The mind-body relationship is evident in various everyday experiences. For instance, stress can lead to physical symptoms such as headaches, muscle tension, and fatigue. Conversely, physical ailments can affect our mental state, leading to anxiety, depression, or a sense of hopelessness. This bidirectional influence highlights the importance of considering both mental and physical aspects in health and well-being.

One of the core principles of the mind-body connection is the concept of psychosomatic responses, where psychological factors can induce or exacerbate physical symptoms. For example, chronic stress can weaken the immune system, making individuals more susceptible to illnesses. Similarly, emotional trauma can manifest as chronic pain or other physical conditions. Understanding this relationship can inform more effective approaches to healthcare, emphasizing the need for treatments that address both mental and physical aspects of health. The mind-body connection also plays a crucial role in the healing process. Practices such as mindfulness meditation, yoga, and tai chi leverage this relationship by promoting mental relaxation and physical well-being. These practices encourage individuals to cultivate awareness of their bodies and minds, fostering a sense of harmony and balance. Research has shown that such mind-body practices can reduce stress, improve mood, and enhance overall health.

The Role of the Nervous System

The nervous system is central to the mind-body connection, serving as the primary communication network between the brain and the rest of the body. It is composed of two main parts: the central nervous system (CNS), which includes the brain and spinal cord, and the peripheral nervous system (PNS), which connects the CNS to the rest of the body.

The autonomic nervous system (ANS), a subdivision of the PNS, plays a critical role in regulating involuntary bodily functions such as heart rate, digestion, and respiratory rate. The ANS is further divided into the sympathetic nervous system (SNS) and the parasympathetic nervous system (PNS), which work together to maintain homeostasis. The sympathetic nervous system is responsible for the "fight or flight" response, which prepares the body to respond to perceived threats. When activated, the SNS increases heart rate, redirects blood flow to essential muscles, and releases stress hormones such as adrenaline and cortisol. This response is essential for survival, enabling quick reactions to danger. However, chronic activation of the SNS, often due to prolonged stress, can lead to negative health outcomes such as hypertension, anxiety, and immune system suppression.

In contrast, the parasympathetic nervous system promotes the "rest and digest" response, which helps the body relax and recover after stress. Activation of the PNS slows the heart rate, enhances digestion, and promotes the release of hormones that facilitate relaxation and healing. A healthy balance between the SNS and PNS is crucial for maintaining overall health and well-being. The nervous system's role in the mind-body connection is further illustrated by its involvement in the stress response. When an individual perceives a threat, the hypothalamus in the brain activates the SNS, triggering a cascade of physiological changes. This response is beneficial in acute situations, but when the stress is chronic, it can lead to long-term health problems.

Understanding the nervous system's role in the mind-body connection can inform strategies to promote balance and resilience. Techniques such as deep breathing, progressive muscle relaxation, and mindfulness meditation can activate the PNS, helping to counteract the effects of chronic stress. By learning to regulate their nervous system responses, individuals can improve their mental and physical health.

How Trauma Affects the Body

Trauma can have profound and lasting effects on the body, often manifesting as physical symptoms and chronic health conditions. When an individual experiences trauma, whether it is physical, emotional, or psychological, the body and mind respond in ways that can leave lasting imprints on their overall well-being. One of the primary ways trauma affects the body is through the activation of the stress response. During a traumatic event, the body's SNS is activated, preparing the individual to either fight, flee, or freeze in response to the threat. This activation involves the release of stress hormones such as adrenaline and cortisol, which facilitate quick physical reactions. While this response is crucial for survival, prolonged or repeated activation due to ongoing trauma can lead to a state of hyperarousal.

Hyperarousal can result in various physical symptoms, including increased heart rate, muscle tension, and heightened sensory awareness. Over time, the constant activation of the stress response can lead to chronic conditions such as hypertension, cardiovascular disease, and digestive disorders. Additionally, the immune system can become compromised, making the individual more susceptible to infections and illnesses. Trauma can also manifest as somatic symptoms, which are physical manifestations of psychological distress. These symptoms can include chronic pain, gastrointestinal issues, and unexplained aches and pains. Somatic symptoms are often the body's way of expressing and coping with unresolved trauma. For many individuals, these symptoms persist long after the traumatic event has ended, serving as a reminder of the past and a source of ongoing distress.

In some cases, trauma can lead to dissociation, a psychological defense mechanism where the individual disconnects from their thoughts, feelings, or bodily sensations. Dissociation can serve as a coping mechanism to protect the individual from overwhelming emotions and memories associated with the trauma. However, it can also lead to a disconnection from the body, making it difficult for individuals to recognize and address their physical needs.

Post-traumatic stress disorder (PTSD) is a condition that exemplifies how trauma can affect the body. Individuals with PTSD may experience flashbacks, nightmares, and intrusive thoughts related to the traumatic event. These psychological symptoms are often accompanied by physical symptoms such as hypervigilance, an exaggerated startle response, and difficulty sleeping. The body's stress response becomes dysregulated, leading to a state of constant alertness and tension. Healing from trauma requires addressing both the psychological and physical aspects of the experience. Somatic therapy, which focuses on the body's role in trauma and healing, can be particularly effective. Techniques such as grounding exercises, body awareness practices, and movement therapy can help individuals release stored trauma and tension from the body. By reconnecting with their bodies and learning to regulate their physiological responses, individuals can begin to heal from the effects of trauma.

The Importance of Body Awareness

Body awareness, also known as interoception, is the ability to perceive and understand the internal sensations of the body. It plays a crucial role in the mind-body connection, as it allows individuals to recognize and respond to their physical needs and emotions. Developing body awareness can lead to improved health, emotional regulation, and overall well-being. One of the key benefits of body awareness is its ability to enhance self-regulation. By tuning into their bodily sensations, individuals can become more attuned to their emotional states and learn to manage their responses to stress and challenges. For example, recognizing the physical signs of stress, such as increased heart rate or muscle tension, can prompt individuals to engage in relaxation techniques or other coping strategies. This awareness can prevent the buildup of chronic stress and its associated health problems.

Body awareness also plays a crucial role in emotional processing. Emotions are often experienced as physical sensations in the body, such as a tight chest, a fluttering stomach, or a lump in the throat. By developing body awareness, individuals can learn to recognize and name these sensations, allowing them to process and express their emotions more effectively. This can lead to improved emotional regulation and a greater sense of emotional balance. In addition to its benefits for emotional health, body awareness can also improve physical health. By tuning into their bodily sensations, individuals can become more aware of their physical needs and take proactive steps to address them. For example, recognizing signs of hunger, fatigue, or discomfort can prompt individuals to eat, rest, or adjust their posture, preventing the development of more serious health issues. Body awareness can also enhance physical performance, as it allows individuals to fine-tune their movements and respond to their body's feedback during physical activities.

Mindfulness practices are a powerful way to develop body awareness. Mindfulness involves paying attention to the present moment with curiosity and non-judgment. By focusing on their bodily sensations, individuals can cultivate a greater sense of connection with their bodies and develop a deeper understanding of their physical and emotional states. Techniques such as body scans, mindful breathing, and mindful movement can help individuals develop this awareness and integrate it into their daily lives. Yoga and other mind-body practices are also effective for enhancing body awareness. These practices involve moving the body with intention and awareness, promoting a sense of embodiment and presence. Through yoga, individuals can learn to listen to their bodies, recognize their limits, and respond to their physical needs with compassion and care. This awareness can extend beyond the yoga mat, influencing how individuals move through their daily lives and interact with their bodies.

Body awareness is also essential for healing from trauma. Traumatic experiences can lead to a disconnection from the body, making it difficult for individuals to recognize and respond to their physical needs. Developing body awareness can help individuals reconnect with their bodies and process their traumatic experiences in a safe and supportive way. Somatic therapy, which emphasizes the body's role in trauma and healing, can be particularly effective for this purpose.

Chapter Three

Getting Started with Somatic Therapy

Somatic therapy is an approach that integrates the mind and body to address physical and psychological symptoms. This holistic method acknowledges the profound connection between emotions and physical experiences, offering a pathway to healing that is grounded in the body's sensations and movements. Whether you are new to somatic therapy or seeking to deepen your practice, understanding the foundational principles and steps involved can significantly enhance your journey toward well-being.

Setting Intentions for Healing

Setting clear intentions is a crucial first step in somatic therapy. Intentions serve as a guiding compass, helping to focus your efforts and energies towards specific healing goals. Begin by reflecting on what you hope to achieve through somatic therapy. Are you looking to release past trauma, reduce stress, improve emotional regulation, or enhance your overall well-being? Identifying your objectives can provide clarity and direction. When setting your intentions, it's important to be both specific and realistic. For instance, instead of a broad goal like "I want to feel better," you might set a more precise intention such as "I want to reduce anxiety during stressful situations." This specificity helps in creating actionable steps and measuring progress. Moreover, be gentle with yourself in this process. Healing is not linear, and it is essential to allow space for gradual improvement and setbacks.

Journaling can be a valuable tool in this stage. Writing down your intentions allows you to articulate your thoughts and feelings clearly. Revisiting these entries periodically can also help you track your progress and adjust your goals as needed. Additionally, sharing your intentions with a therapist or a supportive community can provide further encouragement and accountability.

Creating a Safe Space for Practice

A safe and nurturing environment is fundamental to effective somatic therapy. This space should be physically comfortable and emotionally secure, fostering a sense of safety that allows you to explore and express your inner experiences without fear or judgment. Whether you are practicing at home or in a professional setting, the ambiance of your environment can significantly impact your therapeutic outcomes. Start by selecting a location where you feel most at ease. This could be a quiet room in your home, a peaceful corner in a garden, or a designated therapy space. Ensure that this area is free from distractions and interruptions. Comfort is key, so consider factors like lighting, temperature, and seating arrangements. Soft lighting, a comfortable chair or mat, and a blanket can contribute to a calming atmosphere.

Personalizing your space with items that bring you comfort and joy can also enhance your practice. This might include photographs, plants, essential oils, or soothing music. The goal is to create an environment that feels safe and inviting, allowing you to fully immerse yourself in the therapeutic process. Equally important is the emotional safety of your space. Establish boundaries that protect your time and energy during practice. Inform those around you of your need for uninterrupted time, and consider using a "do not disturb" sign if necessary. Emotional safety also involves self-compassion and patience. Approach your practice with a non-judgmental mindset, acknowledging that all emotions and sensations are valid and worthy of attention.

Tools and Props You May Need

While somatic therapy primarily relies on the body and mind, certain tools and props can enhance the practice and facilitate deeper exploration. These items are not strictly necessary but can provide additional support and comfort. One of the most commonly used props in somatic therapy is a yoga mat or a comfortable rug. This provides a designated space for movement and grounding exercises. Cushions and bolsters can be helpful for maintaining comfortable postures during longer sessions. They can also support the body in restorative poses, aiding relaxation and release.

Other tools that may be beneficial include foam rollers and massage balls, which can be used for self-massage and myofascial release. These tools help to relieve muscle tension and increase body awareness, enhancing the connection between physical sensations and emotional experiences. Breathwork aids such as a breathing cushion or a simple eye mask can also be useful. A breathing cushion supports diaphragmatic breathing, which is a core component of many somatic practices. An eye mask can help to block out visual distractions, allowing for deeper internal focus.

In addition to physical props, consider incorporating sensory items that engage different senses. Aromatherapy with essential oils can create a calming environment, while a sound machine or soft music can provide auditory relaxation. Textured objects like stress balls or tactile fabrics can offer grounding sensations, helping to anchor your attention to the present moment.

Establishing a Routine

Consistency is crucial in somatic therapy, and establishing a regular routine can significantly enhance the benefits of your practice. A well-structured routine provides a sense of stability and continuity, allowing you to build upon each session's progress. Begin by scheduling regular sessions that fit into your daily or weekly routine. Consistency is more important than duration, so even short, frequent sessions can be highly effective. Decide on a time that works best for you, whether it's in the morning to start your day with mindfulness or in the evening to unwind.

Developing a ritual to begin and end your practice can also be beneficial. This might include lighting a candle, playing a specific piece of music, or taking a few moments to center yourself with deep breaths. Rituals help to signal to your mind and body that it is time to transition into a therapeutic space, creating a boundary between your practice and daily life. During your sessions, start with grounding exercises that help you connect with your body. This could involve deep breathing, body scans, or gentle stretching. Grounding exercises prepare your body and mind for deeper work by promoting relaxation and present-moment awareness.

As you progress, incorporate a variety of somatic techniques tailored to your needs and goals. This might include movement practices such as yoga or Tai Chi, expressive arts like dance or drawing, and mindfulness exercises like meditation or guided imagery. Allow your sessions to be fluid and responsive to your current state, adapting your practices based on what feels most supportive. Reflecting on each session can deepen your understanding and integration of the experiences. Take a few minutes to journal or meditate on what you felt, noticed, and learned. This reflection not only consolidates the benefits of your practice but also provides valuable insights for future sessions.

Ultimately, the goal of somatic therapy is to cultivate a deeper connection with your body and emotions, fostering a sense of wholeness and well-being. By setting clear intentions, creating a safe and nurturing environment, utilizing supportive tools, and establishing a consistent routine, you can create a solid foundation for your somatic therapy practice. This holistic approach to healing honors the intricate interplay between mind and body, offering a compassionate pathway to transformation and growth.

Chapter Four

Foundational Techniques for Self-Soothing

Self-soothing techniques are essential skills that help individuals manage stress, anxiety, and other emotional challenges. By cultivating these techniques, one can foster a sense of inner calm and resilience, enabling better emotional regulation and overall well-being. Understanding and integrating foundational self-soothing methods can provide valuable tools for navigating life's ups and downs with greater ease and confidence.

Grounding Techniques

Grounding techniques are practical methods designed to anchor an individual in the present moment. These techniques are especially useful during periods of intense stress, anxiety, or dissociation, as they help to shift focus from distressing thoughts and emotions to the here and now. Grounding can involve physical, mental, or sensory strategies, each aiming to create a sense of stability and control. One effective grounding technique is the 5-4-3-2-1 method. This involves identifying five things you can see, four things you can touch, three things you can hear, two things you can smell, and one thing you can taste. This exercise engages multiple senses, redirecting attention away from anxiety or distressing thoughts and into the immediate environment. The process of naming these items helps to interrupt negative thought patterns and promote a sense of presence.

Another grounding strategy is the use of physical sensation. This can include activities such as walking barefoot on grass, holding a piece of ice, or taking a cold shower. The physical sensations associated with these activities can be incredibly grounding, bringing attention back to the body and the present moment. Similarly, engaging in rhythmic movements like tapping your feet, clenching and unclenching your fists, or even swaying can provide a grounding effect.

Mental grounding techniques can also be highly effective. These might involve simple mental exercises such as counting backward from 100 by sevens, reciting a favorite poem or song lyrics, or visualizing a safe and peaceful place. These mental activities require concentration, which helps to divert focus away from distressing emotions and thoughts. Visualizations, in particular, can create a powerful sense of safety and calm by mentally transporting you to a place where you feel secure and at ease. Grounding techniques are versatile and can be adapted to suit individual preferences and contexts. The key is to find methods that resonate personally and can be easily implemented in moments of need. Practicing these techniques regularly can also enhance their effectiveness, making them more accessible during times of heightened stress or anxiety.

Breathing Exercises

Breathing exercises are a cornerstone of self-soothing practices. Controlled breathing can significantly impact the autonomic nervous system, promoting relaxation and reducing stress. By focusing on breath, individuals can calm their minds and bodies, creating a sense of tranquility and balance. One of the simplest and most effective breathing exercises is diaphragmatic breathing, also known as belly breathing. This technique involves breathing deeply into the abdomen rather than the chest. To practice, sit or lie down in a comfortable position, place one hand on your chest and the other on your abdomen. Inhale deeply through your nose, allowing your abdomen to rise as it fills with air. Exhale slowly through your mouth, letting your abdomen fall. This deep, slow breathing pattern activates the parasympathetic nervous system, which is responsible for the body's rest-and-digest functions, thereby reducing stress and promoting relaxation.

Another powerful breathing exercise is the 4-7-8 technique, developed by Dr. Andrew Weil. This method involves inhaling for a count of four, holding the breath for a count of seven, and exhaling for a count of eight. This extended exhalation helps to expel more carbon dioxide from the lungs, slowing the heart rate and promoting a state of calm. Practicing this technique regularly can enhance its soothing effects and improve overall respiratory efficiency.

Box breathing, also known as square breathing, is another effective method. This technique involves inhaling for a count of four, holding the breath for a count of four, exhaling for a count of four, and holding the breath again for a count of four. The repetitive, rhythmic nature of box breathing can help to regulate the breath and create a sense of balance and stability. This method is particularly useful in high-stress situations, as it provides a structured approach to calming the mind and body.

Alternate nostril breathing, or Nadi Shodhana, is a technique rooted in yoga and Ayurvedic traditions. This practice involves breathing through one nostril at a time, alternating between the left and right nostrils. To practice, sit comfortably, use your right thumb to close your right nostril, and inhale deeply through your left nostril. Close your left nostril with your right ring finger, release your thumb from your right nostril, and exhale through the right nostril. Inhale through the right nostril, close it with your thumb, and exhale through the left nostril. This cycle can be repeated several times. Alternate nostril breathing helps to balance the hemispheres of the brain, reduce stress, and promote a sense of overall well-being.

Progressive Muscle Relaxation

Progressive muscle relaxation (PMR) is a technique that involves systematically tensing and then relaxing different muscle groups in the body. This method helps to reduce physical tension and promote relaxation, making it an effective tool for managing stress and anxiety. To practice PMR, find a quiet and comfortable place where you can sit or lie down. Begin by focusing on your breathing, taking a few deep breaths to center yourself. Start with your feet, tensing the muscles in your toes and feet as tightly as you can. Hold the tension for a few seconds, then release it, allowing the muscles to relax completely. Notice the difference between the feeling of tension and relaxation. Move up to your calves, repeating the process of tensing and relaxing. Continue this practice, progressing through your thighs, abdomen, chest, arms, and face, until you have tensed and relaxed all major muscle groups.

The goal of PMR is to increase awareness of physical tension and learn to release it. By intentionally tensing and then relaxing the muscles, you can develop a heightened sense of bodily awareness and a greater ability to recognize and reduce tension in everyday life. Regular practice of PMR can also improve sleep, reduce symptoms of anxiety, and enhance overall physical and mental relaxation. For individuals new to PMR, guided recordings or scripts can be particularly helpful. These resources provide step-by-step instructions, guiding you through each muscle group and ensuring that you maintain a slow and steady pace. As you become more familiar with the technique, you can adapt the practice to suit your needs, focusing on specific areas of tension or incorporating PMR into your daily routine.

Sensory Awareness Practices

Sensory awareness practices involve engaging and enhancing the senses to promote relaxation and mindfulness. These practices help to anchor attention in the present moment, reduce stress, and foster a deeper connection with the body and environment. One effective sensory awareness practice is mindful eating. This involves paying close attention to the sensory experiences of eating, such as the taste, texture, smell, and appearance of food. Begin by selecting a small piece of food, such as a raisin or a piece of chocolate. Observe its color, shape, and texture. Smell the food, noticing any aromas. Place the food in your mouth, but before chewing, take a moment to feel its texture. Slowly chew, paying attention to the flavors and sensations. This mindful approach to eating can transform a routine activity into a meditative practice, enhancing enjoyment and promoting a sense of presence.

Another sensory practice is the use of aromatherapy. Essential oils, such as lavender, chamomile, or eucalyptus, can be used to create a calming environment. Diffusing these oils in your space or adding a few drops to a warm bath can help to soothe the senses and promote relaxation. Inhaling these scents can trigger the brain's limbic system, which is involved in emotion regulation and stress response, thereby enhancing mood and reducing anxiety. Listening to music or nature sounds is also a powerful sensory practice. Choose music that resonates with you, whether it's classical, jazz, ambient, or any other genre that you find soothing. Alternatively, listening to nature sounds like ocean waves, rain, or birdsong can create a peaceful auditory environment. Close your eyes and focus on the sounds, allowing them to wash over you and bring a sense of calm. This practice can be especially helpful for unwinding at the end of the day or creating a relaxing atmosphere during stressful times.

Engaging in tactile activities can also enhance sensory awareness and promote relaxation. This might include activities like knitting, playing with clay or sand, or simply running your hands over different textures like soft fabric or smooth stones. The physical sensations associated with these activities can be grounding and calming, helping to shift focus away from stress and into the present moment. Visual sensory practices, such as creating or viewing art, can also be deeply soothing. Drawing, painting, or coloring can provide an outlet for expression and relaxation. Alternatively, simply observing art or nature can be calming. Spend time in a garden, park, or any natural setting, and take in the colors, shapes, and movements around you. Allowing yourself to be visually immersed in beauty can reduce stress and promote a sense of peace.

Incorporating sensory awareness practices into your daily routine can enhance overall well-being and provide a reliable toolkit for managing stress. By regularly engaging the senses in mindful and intentional ways, you can cultivate a deeper connection with yourself and the world around you, fostering a sense of balance and harmony.

Chapter Five

Techniques for Trauma Release

Trauma, whether from a single event or a series of prolonged experiences, can deeply affect both the mind and body. The impacts of trauma often manifest in various forms, including anxiety, depression, physical pain, and emotional dysregulation. To address and heal these effects, various techniques for trauma release have been developed, focusing on reconnecting the mind and body, releasing stored tension, and fostering a sense of safety and empowerment. Understanding these techniques and their applications can provide a comprehensive approach to healing from trauma.

Understanding Trauma Responses

To effectively address trauma, it is crucial to understand the body's responses to traumatic experiences. Trauma responses are the body's natural reactions to perceived threats, which are deeply rooted in our physiology. The autonomic nervous system (ANS) plays a central role in these responses, particularly through its sympathetic and parasympathetic branches. When faced with danger, the sympathetic nervous system triggers the fight-or-flight response, preparing the body to either confront or escape the threat. This response involves a cascade of physiological changes, including increased heart rate, heightened alertness, and the release of stress hormones like adrenaline and cortisol.

However, when a threat is perceived as inescapable or overwhelming, the body may enter a state of freeze, mediated by the parasympathetic nervous system. In this state, the body essentially shuts down, leading to feelings of numbness, immobility, and disconnection. While these responses are adaptive survival mechanisms, they can become maladaptive if they persist long after the threat has passed. Chronic activation of these responses can lead to a range of symptoms, including hypervigilance, flashbacks, emotional numbness, and difficulties with concentration and sleep.

Understanding these trauma responses is the first step in addressing them. Recognizing that these responses are natural and automatic can help individuals approach their healing with compassion and patience. By learning to identify and work with these responses, individuals can begin to release the physiological and emotional tension associated with trauma, paving the way for healing and recovery.

Shaking and Tremoring for Release

One of the most natural and effective techniques for trauma release is shaking and tremoring. These involuntary movements are the body's way of discharging excess energy and tension accumulated during a traumatic event. In the animal kingdom, it is common to see animals shake or tremble after a threat has passed, effectively releasing the built-up stress and returning to a state of calm. Humans, however, often suppress these natural impulses, leading to the retention of tension and trauma in the body.

Trauma Release Exercises (TRE), developed by Dr. David Berceli, are a series of exercises designed to elicit these natural shaking and tremoring responses. TRE involves a sequence of physical movements that fatigue specific muscle groups, particularly in the legs and hips, which are then followed by a period of lying down to allow the body to tremor. This tremoring process helps to release deep-seated tension and reset the nervous system.

To practice TRE, begin with a warm-up to gently stretch and prepare the body. Next, perform a series of exercises that involve sustained postures and slight movements to fatigue the muscles. For example, standing with knees slightly bent and holding this position can create the necessary muscle fatigue. After completing the exercises, lie down on your back with your knees bent and feet flat on the floor. Allow your legs to gently move from side to side or up and down, facilitating the natural tremoring response. Focus on your breath and observe the sensations in your body without trying to control or suppress the movements. Shaking and tremoring can also occur spontaneously in other contexts, such as during yoga, dance, or other physical activities. Allowing these movements to happen naturally, without judgment or suppression, can be highly beneficial. It is important to approach this practice with a sense of safety and self-compassion, ensuring that the environment is secure and that you are emotionally ready to engage with the release process.

Using Movement for Healing

Movement is a powerful tool for trauma healing, as it helps to reconnect the mind and body, release stored tension, and promote a sense of empowerment and agency. Various forms of movement, such as yoga, dance, and somatic experiencing, can be particularly effective in addressing trauma.

Yoga, for instance, combines physical postures, breathwork, and mindfulness to create a holistic approach to healing. Trauma-sensitive yoga, a specialized form of yoga developed to support trauma survivors, emphasizes safety, choice, and mindfulness. This approach avoids triggering postures or language and encourages participants to listen to their bodies and move at their own pace. Through gentle and mindful movement, individuals can begin to reconnect with their bodies, release tension, and cultivate a sense of inner calm and safety.

Dance and expressive movement also offer powerful avenues for trauma healing. Dance Movement Therapy (DMT) is a therapeutic practice that uses movement and dance to promote emotional, cognitive, and physical integration. In DMT, individuals are encouraged to express their emotions and experiences through movement, allowing for the release of pent-up tension and fostering a sense of self-expression and empowerment. Improvised and free-form dance can also be highly therapeutic, providing a space for spontaneous and uninhibited movement that can help to release stored emotions and promote a sense of freedom and joy.

Somatic Experiencing (SE), developed by Dr. Peter Levine, is a body-oriented approach to trauma healing that focuses on the felt sense of the body. SE practitioners guide individuals in tuning into their bodily sensations and using movement to release tension and restore balance to the nervous system. This approach emphasizes the importance of completing the body's natural defensive responses, such as running or fighting, which may have been interrupted during the traumatic event. By gently guiding the body through these movements, SE helps to release trapped energy and promote healing. Incorporating movement into daily life can also support trauma healing. Simple activities such as walking, stretching, or gentle exercise can help to release tension and promote a sense of well-being. The key is to move in ways that feel safe and enjoyable, allowing the body to guide the process. Regular movement practices can help to build resilience, enhance body awareness, and support overall mental and physical health.

Safe Touch and Self-Holding

Touch is a fundamental aspect of human experience and can play a significant role in trauma healing. Safe, nurturing touch can help to soothe the nervous system, foster a sense of connection and safety, and promote healing. However, for trauma survivors, physical touch can sometimes be triggering or overwhelming. It is essential to approach touch with sensitivity and care, ensuring that it is always consensual and respectful of individual boundaries. Safe touch can come from a trusted therapist, partner, or even from oneself. In therapeutic settings, touch should always be discussed and agreed upon beforehand, with clear boundaries and consent. Techniques such as therapeutic massage, Reiki, or craniosacral therapy can provide gentle and supportive touch that helps to release tension and promote relaxation.

Self-holding and self-touch can also be powerful tools for trauma healing. These techniques involve using one's own hands to provide comforting and grounding touch to different parts of the body. For example, placing a hand on the heart and another on the abdomen can create a sense of safety and connection. Gently holding the sides of the face, cradling the back of the head, or wrapping the arms around the body in a self-hug can also be deeply soothing.

To practice self-holding, find a quiet and comfortable space where you can sit or lie down. Begin by taking a few deep breaths to center yourself. Place your hands on a part of your body that feels comforting, such as your heart, abdomen, or face. Apply gentle pressure, as if you were comforting a loved one. Focus on the sensations of warmth and contact, allowing yourself to feel supported and cared for. You can also use words of affirmation or self-compassion, silently or aloud, to enhance the sense of nurturing and safety.

In addition to self-holding, incorporating sensory elements can enhance the soothing effects of touch. Using a weighted blanket, soft fabrics, or textured objects can provide additional sensory input that promotes relaxation and grounding. These elements can help to create a multisensory experience that supports the body's natural healing processes. Touch and self-holding techniques can be integrated into daily routines as part of a broader self-care practice. Taking time each day to engage in comforting touch, whether through self-massage, gentle stretching, or simply resting a hand on the heart, can help to build resilience and support emotional well-being. It is essential to approach these practices with mindfulness and self-compassion, honoring your body's needs and boundaries.

Chapter Six

Building Mind-Body Balance

Building mind-body balance involves integrating practices that enhance the connection between mental and physical well-being. This holistic approach recognizes the interconnectedness of the mind and body, emphasizing practices that promote harmony, resilience, and overall health. By cultivating awareness, mindfulness, and intentional movement, individuals can foster a deeper understanding of themselves and create a foundation for sustained well-being.

Mindful Movement Practices

Mindful movement practices are forms of physical activity that emphasize awareness of the body and present-moment experience. These practices combine movement with mindfulness techniques such as deep breathing, focused attention, and non-judgmental awareness. By integrating mindfulness into movement, individuals can enhance physical fitness while also promoting mental clarity, stress reduction, and emotional regulation.

Tai Chi and Qigong are ancient Chinese practices that exemplify mindful movement. Tai Chi consists of slow, deliberate movements that flow seamlessly from one to the next, accompanied by deep breathing and focused attention. Qigong, on the other hand, involves gentle movements, postures, and breathing exercises designed to cultivate and balance qi (life energy) within the body. Both practices emphasize relaxation, balance, and the cultivation of inner peace.

Another popular mindful movement practice is Pilates, which focuses on core strength, flexibility, and posture. Pilates exercises are performed with controlled breathing and precise movements, emphasizing alignment and awareness of body mechanics. This mindful approach helps individuals develop body awareness, improve coordination, and alleviate muscular imbalances.

Walking meditation is a simple yet profound mindful movement practice that can be practiced anywhere. During walking meditation, attention is focused on the sensations of walking—such as the movement of the feet, the rhythm of the breath, and the environment around you. This practice encourages mindfulness in motion, fostering a sense of groundedness and presence in each step. Mindful movement practices offer numerous benefits for mind-body balance. Regular practice can improve physical fitness, enhance flexibility and strength, reduce stress and anxiety, and promote overall well-being. By cultivating mindfulness through movement, individuals can deepen their connection to their bodies, increase self-awareness, and develop resilience in the face of life's challenges.

Yoga for Somatic Healing

Yoga is a holistic practice that integrates physical postures (asanas), breathwork (pranayama), and meditation to promote health and well-being. Originating in ancient India, yoga has evolved into various styles and approaches, each offering unique benefits for mind-body balance and healing. When applied with a somatic focus, yoga becomes a powerful tool for releasing tension, cultivating body awareness, and supporting emotional resilience. Somatic yoga emphasizes the felt sense of the body and encourages individuals to explore sensations, movements, and breath in a mindful way. This approach helps to release physical and emotional tension stored in the body, promoting relaxation and restoring balance to the nervous system. By practicing yoga somatically, individuals can develop a deeper understanding of their bodies and their unique needs for healing and self-care.

Restorative yoga is another gentle and nurturing style that focuses on relaxation and deep rest. In restorative yoga, passive postures are held for extended periods, supported by props such as bolsters, blankets, and blocks. This allows the body to release tension and stress, promoting a state of deep relaxation and rejuvenation. Restorative yoga is particularly beneficial for individuals recovering from illness or injury, as well as those experiencing chronic stress or fatigue.

Yin yoga is a slow-paced style that targets the connective tissues of the body, such as ligaments, tendons, and fascia. In Yin yoga, postures are held for longer durations—typically three to five minutes or more—allowing for deep stretching and release. This practice helps to increase flexibility, improve joint mobility, and release tension stored deep within the body. Yin yoga also cultivates mindfulness and introspection, as practitioners are encouraged to observe sensations and emotions that arise during practice. Practicing yoga for somatic healing involves creating a safe and supportive environment for exploration and self-discovery. It is essential to approach yoga with compassion and non-judgment, honoring the body's limitations and embracing the present moment experience. By integrating breath, movement, and mindfulness, yoga becomes a transformative practice that promotes holistic healing and fosters mind-body balance.

Dance and Expressive Movement

Dance and expressive movement offer powerful avenues for self-expression, emotional release, and mind-body integration. Through movement, individuals can access and process emotions, memories, and experiences that may be difficult to articulate verbally. Dance therapy, also known as Dance Movement Therapy (DMT), is a specialized form of psychotherapy that uses movement and dance to promote emotional, cognitive, and physical integration. In DMT sessions, individuals are invited to explore and express themselves through movement, guided by a trained therapist. This approach allows for the embodiment of feelings and experiences, fostering self-awareness and insight. DMT techniques may include improvisation, structured movement sequences, and creative expression through dance. By engaging in expressive movement, individuals can release pent-up emotions, reduce stress, and cultivate a sense of empowerment and self-confidence.

Ecstatic dance is another form of expressive movement that emphasizes free-form, spontaneous dancing to rhythmic music. In ecstatic dance sessions, participants are encouraged to move intuitively, without judgment or inhibition. This practice promotes self-expression, creativity, and connection with others in a supportive and non-verbal environment. Ecstatic dance can be deeply cathartic, allowing individuals to release tension, uplift their spirits, and experience a sense of freedom and joy through movement. Integrating dance and expressive movement into daily life can support mind-body balance and emotional well-being. Dancing alone or with others can be a joyful way to release stress, boost mood, and increase energy levels. Moving the body rhythmically to music also stimulates the release of endorphins—natural mood-enhancing chemicals in the brain—that promote feelings of happiness and relaxation.

Integrating Breath with Movement

Integrating breath with movement is a core principle in many mind-body practices, enhancing the effectiveness of physical exercises and promoting mindfulness and relaxation. Breathwork techniques such as deep breathing, synchronized breathing, and breath awareness help to regulate the nervous system, calm the mind, and deepen the mind-body connection. In yoga, the coordination of breath and movement is known as vinyasa or flow. Vinyasa yoga classes typically involve a series of postures linked together in a flowing sequence, with each movement synchronized with either an inhalation or exhalation. This mindful approach to yoga not only enhances physical flexibility and strength but also promotes mental focus and relaxation. By coordinating breath with movement, practitioners can cultivate a sense of fluidity and mindfulness in their practice.

Pilates also emphasizes the importance of breath control and coordination. In Pilates exercises, breath is used to initiate and support movements, promoting core stability, alignment, and efficient movement patterns. Deep diaphragmatic breathing engages the parasympathetic nervous system, promoting relaxation and reducing stress. By integrating breath with movement, Pilates practitioners can enhance body awareness, improve posture, and support overall well-being.

Tai Chi and Qigong similarly incorporate breathwork to enhance the flow of qi (life energy) within the body. These practices emphasize slow, deliberate movements coordinated with deep abdominal breathing. By focusing on the breath, practitioners can cultivate a calm and centered state of mind, harmonize the body's energy systems, and promote physical and emotional balance.

Integrating breath with movement can be applied to everyday activities as well, enhancing mindfulness and promoting relaxation in various contexts. Simple practices such as walking with synchronized breath, practicing mindful stretching, or engaging in gentle exercise routines can help individuals stay present, reduce stress, and enhance overall well-being. By cultivating awareness of breath and its connection to physical movement, individuals can harness the transformative power of mind-body integration to support their health and vitality.

Chapter Seven

Techniques for Resilience Building

Resilience, the ability to bounce back from adversity, is a crucial skill that can be developed and strengthened throughout life. Techniques for resilience building encompass a variety of strategies aimed at enhancing emotional strength, fostering a resilient core self, establishing supportive networks, and integrating daily practices that promote resilience.

Developing Emotional Resilience

Emotional resilience involves the capacity to adapt to stressful situations, manage emotions effectively, and maintain a sense of perspective amidst challenges. One key technique for developing emotional resilience is cultivating mindfulness. Mindfulness practices, such as meditation and mindful breathing, help individuals observe their thoughts and emotions without judgment.

This awareness allows for better emotional regulation and reduces reactivity in stressful situations.

Another effective technique is cognitive restructuring, which involves identifying and challenging negative thought patterns. By replacing irrational or catastrophic thoughts with more balanced and realistic ones, individuals can build a more resilient mindset. Additionally, practicing self-compassion—being kind and understanding toward oneself during difficult times—fosters resilience by promoting emotional healing and reducing self-criticism.

Physical well-being also plays a crucial role in emotional resilience. Regular exercise, adequate sleep, and healthy nutrition contribute to overall resilience by reducing stress levels, improving mood, and enhancing cognitive function. Engaging in hobbies and activities that bring joy and fulfillment further supports emotional resilience by fostering a sense of purpose and satisfaction.

Strengthening the Core Self

Strengthening the core self involves cultivating a strong sense of identity, values, and purpose that serve as anchors during challenging times. Self-awareness is a fundamental aspect of this process, as it allows individuals to understand their strengths, weaknesses, and personal boundaries. Journaling, introspection, and self-reflection exercises can facilitate deeper self-awareness and strengthen the core self.

Setting meaningful goals aligned with personal values and aspirations provides direction and motivation, even in the face of setbacks. Goal-setting techniques, such as SMART goals (Specific, Measurable, Achievable, Relevant, Time-bound), help individuals break down larger objectives into smaller, manageable steps. Celebrating progress and achievements along the way reinforces self-confidence and resilience.

Practicing authenticity—being true to oneself and honoring one's values—builds a resilient core self by fostering inner integrity and self-respect. This involves making choices and decisions that align with personal beliefs and principles, even when facing external pressures or challenges. Building resilience also entails embracing life's uncertainties and learning from failures or setbacks, which contribute to personal growth and resilience over time.

Building a Support System

Building a support system is essential for resilience, as social connections provide emotional validation, practical assistance, and a sense of belonging. Cultivating supportive relationships with family, friends, peers, or mentors involves nurturing trust, empathy, and mutual respect. Effective communication skills, such as active listening and assertiveness, enhance relationship quality and strengthen the support network.

Seeking professional support from counselors, therapists, or support groups can also be beneficial, especially during times of significant stress or adversity. These resources provide guidance, perspective, and therapeutic interventions that promote emotional healing and resilience building. Building a diverse support network that includes both personal and professional connections ensures access to multiple sources of support and perspective.

Engaging in community activities, volunteer work, or group hobbies fosters a sense of community and belonging, which contributes to resilience. Participation in shared interests or causes allows individuals to connect with others who share similar values or experiences, fostering mutual support and solidarity. Building resilience through community involvement also promotes a sense of purpose and contribution to the greater good.

Practices for Daily Resilience

Practices for daily resilience involve integrating habits and routines that support emotional well-being, stress management, and adaptive coping strategies. Establishing a daily routine that includes time for self-care, relaxation, and mindfulness promotes consistency and stability, which are foundational aspects of resilience. Prioritizing self-care activities such as exercise, healthy eating, adequate sleep, and relaxation techniques enhances physical and emotional resilience.

Mindfulness practices, such as meditation, mindful breathing, or body scans, can be integrated into daily routines to promote present-moment awareness and reduce stress. These practices cultivate a calm and centered mindset, enabling individuals to respond to challenges with greater clarity and resilience. Incorporating gratitude practices, such as keeping a gratitude journal or expressing appreciation for others, fosters a positive outlook and resilience by focusing on strengths and blessings.

Engaging in creative outlets, hobbies, or recreational activities provides opportunities for self-expression, enjoyment, and stress relief. Creative pursuits, such as art, music, writing, or gardening, promote emotional well-being by allowing individuals to channel emotions, explore new interests, and recharge their energy. Maintaining a balanced lifestyle that includes time for work, leisure, socializing, and relaxation supports overall resilience and prevents burnout.

Chapter Eight

Advanced Somatic Techniques

Advanced somatic techniques represent a specialized approach to healing that integrates the body and mind, focusing on the interconnection between physical sensations, emotions, and psychological well-being. These approaches are rooted in the understanding that traumatic experiences and chronic stress can become stored in the body, impacting overall health and functioning. By addressing these somatic (body-based) aspects of trauma and stress, these techniques aim to facilitate healing, enhance resilience, and promote holistic well-being.

Somatic Experiencing

Somatic Experiencing (SE), developed by Dr. Peter Levine, is a body-oriented approach designed to address and heal trauma-related symptoms and stress disorders. Central to SE is the understanding that trauma overwhelms the nervous system's natural ability to regulate arousal states. During traumatic events, the body's instinctive fight-flight-freeze responses can become dysregulated, leaving the individual stuck in a state of heightened arousal or numbing.

The SE approach focuses on guiding individuals through a process of titration and pendulation—gradually and safely exploring traumatic memories and bodily sensations. Through gentle tracking of physical sensations and emotional experiences, SE helps individuals renegotiate and complete these defensive responses that were interrupted during the traumatic event. This process allows for the discharge of stored energy associated with trauma, promoting relaxation, restoring nervous system balance, and facilitating emotional healing.

SE sessions typically involve creating a safe therapeutic environment where clients can explore and process sensations and emotions at their own pace. Practitioners trained in SE use gentle interventions to support clients in developing greater tolerance for physical and emotional experiences, thereby promoting resilience and well-being. By fostering a deepened awareness of bodily sensations and facilitating the release of stored tension, SE helps individuals reclaim a sense of safety, empowerment, and agency in their lives.

Bioenergetic Analysis

Bioenergetic Analysis combines insights from psychoanalysis with body-oriented techniques to promote emotional release, physical expression, and increased bioenergy flow. Developed by Alexander Lowen and John Pierrakos, Bioenergetic Analysis posits that muscular tension and blocks in the body can inhibit emotional and psychological well-being. These tensions often reflect unconscious defenses and unresolved emotions stored in the body.

Key techniques in Bioenergetic Analysis include body awareness exercises, breathing techniques, and specific physical movements designed to release muscular tension and promote emotional expression. Practitioners trained in Bioenergetic Analysis help clients explore and release chronic patterns of muscular holding and tension, which can be associated with past traumas or ongoing stressors.

Sessions typically begin with an assessment of bodily tensions and postural habits that may reflect emotional and psychological states. Through guided interventions such as grounding exercises, expressive movements, and verbal processing, clients are encouraged to deepen their awareness of bodily sensations and emotions. Bioenergetic Analysis emphasizes the integration of body and mind, fostering a holistic approach to healing that supports personal growth, emotional resilience, and increased vitality.

Integrative Body-Mind Training

Integrative Body-Mind Training (IBMT) is a mindfulness-based practice that integrates Eastern contemplative traditions with modern therapeutic approaches. Originating from ancient Chinese meditation practices, IBMT emphasizes the interaction between cognitive, emotional, and physical processes to promote well-being and resilience. This approach seeks to optimize the balance and integration of mind-body functions through mindfulness training and body-awareness techniques.

IBMT sessions typically involve guided mindfulness practices that cultivate relaxation, focused attention, and awareness of bodily sensations. Practitioners trained in IBMT help clients develop skills in observing thoughts and sensations without attachment or judgment, fostering a state of mental clarity and emotional balance. By cultivating present-moment awareness and enhancing self-regulation skills, IBMT supports resilience to stress and promotes adaptive coping strategies.

Research on IBMT has demonstrated its effectiveness in improving attentional control, emotional regulation, and physiological health indicators such as heart rate variability and cortisol levels. By integrating mindfulness with body-oriented techniques such as posture adjustment and relaxation, IBMT offers a holistic approach to enhancing overall well-being and promoting resilience in the face of life's challenges.

Somatic Meditation Practices

Somatic meditation practices integrate mindfulness meditation with a focus on bodily sensations, movement, and posture. These practices emphasize the embodiment of mindfulness—bringing awareness to physical sensations, emotions, and the interplay between body and mind. Drawing from traditions such as Tibetan Buddhism, Taoism, and contemporary somatic psychology, somatic meditation offers diverse approaches to deepening self-awareness and promoting holistic healing.

Body scan meditation is a foundational somatic practice that involves systematically scanning the body from head to toe, noticing and releasing tension or discomfort. This practice cultivates body awareness, relaxation, and a grounded presence in the present moment. By directing attention to different parts of the body and observing sensations without judgment, individuals can develop greater self-awareness and resilience to stress.

Walking meditation is another somatic technique that encourages mindfulness during movement. Practitioners synchronize breath awareness with each step taken, cultivating a sense of embodied presence and inner calm. Dynamic movement practices, such as Qi Gong or Feldenkrais Method, combine mindful awareness with gentle physical movements to promote flexibility, balance, and energy flow throughout the body. Incorporating somatic meditation practices into daily life provides opportunities to cultivate mindfulness, enhance self-awareness, and deepen the mind-body connection. By integrating mindfulness with bodily awareness, individuals can develop resilience to stress, improve emotional regulation, and promote overall health and vitality. Somatic meditation offers a pathway to healing and personal growth by honoring the wisdom of the body and nurturing holistic well-being.

Chapter Nine

Combining Somatic Therapy with Other Modalities

Integrating Somatic Therapy with Cognitive Behavioral Therapy (CBT)

Integrating Somatic Therapy with Cognitive Behavioral Therapy (CBT) represents a comprehensive approach to addressing both the physiological and cognitive-emotional aspects of mental health and well-being. CBT focuses on identifying and modifying dysfunctional thought patterns and behaviors that contribute to psychological distress, while Somatic Therapy emphasizes the connection between bodily sensations, emotions, and trauma. Combining these modalities allows for a holistic treatment approach that targets both the mind and body. In practice, integrating Somatic Therapy with CBT involves recognizing how bodily sensations and physiological responses can influence thoughts, emotions, and behaviors. Somatic techniques such as body scanning, breath awareness, and grounding exercises can be incorporated into CBT sessions to help clients deepen their awareness of physical sensations associated with stress, anxiety, or trauma triggers. By exploring these bodily responses, clients gain insight into the interplay between their thoughts, emotions, and bodily experiences.

CBT techniques, such as cognitive restructuring and behavioral experiments, complement somatic interventions by addressing cognitive distortions and promoting adaptive coping strategies. For example, a client experiencing panic attacks may benefit from CBT techniques to challenge catastrophic thoughts while simultaneously learning somatic techniques to regulate physiological arousal and promote relaxation. Collaboration between Somatic Therapists and CBT practitioners enhances treatment outcomes by offering clients a comprehensive toolkit for managing symptoms, improving emotional regulation, and fostering resilience. This integrative approach acknowledges the interconnected nature of mind and body, promoting healing on multiple levels and supporting long-term recovery.

Using Somatic Practices in Mindfulness and Meditation

Using Somatic Practices in Mindfulness and Meditation combines the principles of somatic awareness with traditional contemplative practices to enhance self-awareness, emotional regulation, and overall well-being. Mindfulness meditation involves cultivating present-moment awareness and non-judgmental acceptance of thoughts, emotions, and bodily sensations. Somatic practices, such as body scan meditation, mindful movement, or somatic experiencing techniques, deepen mindfulness practice by integrating attention to physical sensations and the felt experience of emotions.

Body scan meditation, a foundational somatic practice, guides practitioners through a systematic exploration of bodily sensations from head to toe. This practice promotes relaxation, body awareness, and a grounded presence in the present moment. By directing attention to different parts of the body and observing sensations without judgment, individuals develop greater self-awareness and resilience to stress.

Mindful movement practices, such as yoga, Tai Chi, or Qigong, integrate breath awareness with gentle physical movements to promote flexibility, balance, and energy flow throughout the body. These practices cultivate mindfulness in motion, enhancing body-mind integration and supporting emotional regulation and stress reduction.

Somatic experiencing techniques, developed by Dr. Peter Levine, focus on releasing physical tension and stored trauma through gentle exploration of bodily sensations and movements. Integrating these techniques into mindfulness and meditation practices allows individuals to deepen their understanding of the mind-body connection, heal from past trauma, and cultivate resilience and inner peace. By using somatic practices in mindfulness and meditation, individuals can enhance their capacity for self-regulation, emotional resilience, and overall well-being. These integrated approaches offer diverse pathways to healing, personal growth, and spiritual development, fostering a deeper connection with oneself and the world.

The Role of Nutrition and Somatic Health

The Role of Nutrition and Somatic Health underscores the importance of dietary choices and nutritional support in promoting optimal physical and mental well-being. Somatic health refers to the integration of bodily sensations, emotions, and physiological processes that influence overall health and vitality. Nutrition plays a crucial role in supporting somatic health by providing essential nutrients, energy, and biochemical substances necessary for cellular function, brain health, and emotional regulation.

A balanced diet rich in whole foods, fruits, vegetables, lean proteins, and healthy fats supports optimal brain function and neurotransmitter balance, which are essential for mood regulation and stress management. Nutritional deficiencies or imbalances can contribute to physical symptoms such as fatigue, irritability, and digestive disturbances, affecting overall somatic health and emotional well-being. Certain nutrients play specific roles in supporting mental health and somatic functioning. For example, omega-3 fatty acids found in fish oil and flaxseed are crucial for brain health and mood regulation. B vitamins, magnesium, and zinc are involved in neurotransmitter synthesis and cellular energy production, influencing cognitive function and emotional stability.

The gut-brain connection highlights the relationship between gut health, microbiome diversity, and mental well-being. The gut microbiota produce neurotransmitters such as serotonin and gamma-aminobutyric acid (GABA), which play key roles in mood regulation and stress response. A balanced diet that supports gut health—such as consuming probiotic-rich foods, fiber, and prebiotics—can enhance somatic health and promote emotional resilience. Incorporating mindful eating practices—such as paying attention to hunger and fullness cues, savoring flavors, and practicing gratitude for nourishing foods—supports a positive relationship with food and enhances somatic awareness. Mindful eating encourages individuals to make conscious food choices that align with their nutritional needs and support overall health and well-being.

The role of nutrition in somatic health extends beyond physical nourishment to encompass emotional and psychological aspects of well-being. By prioritizing a balanced diet, individuals can support their somatic health, enhance resilience to stress, and promote overall vitality and emotional well-being.

Working with a Professional Therapist

Working with a Professional Therapist provides a structured and supportive environment for individuals seeking to address mental health concerns, navigate life transitions, or enhance personal growth. Professional therapists, including licensed counselors, psychologists, social workers, and psychiatrists, are trained to assess and treat a wide range of emotional, behavioral, and relational issues using evidence-based approaches.

Choosing a therapist who integrates somatic therapy techniques ensures a holistic approach to treatment that considers the interconnected nature of mind, body, and emotions. Somatic therapists are trained to help clients explore and process physical sensations, emotions, and trauma responses stored in the body. Through guided interventions such as body awareness exercises, breathwork, and gentle movement, somatic therapists support clients in developing greater self-awareness, emotional regulation, and resilience.

Therapy sessions provide a safe and confidential space for clients to explore their thoughts, feelings, and experiences without judgment. Therapists use a collaborative approach to develop personalized treatment plans that address individual needs, goals, and strengths. Integrating somatic therapy with other modalities, such as cognitive-behavioral therapy (CBT), mindfulness practices, or nutritional counseling, enhances the therapeutic process by offering diverse tools and strategies for healing and growth.

Effective therapy involves building a trusting therapeutic relationship based on empathy, respect, and confidentiality. Therapists create a supportive environment where clients feel heard, understood, and empowered to explore and resolve challenges. By working with a professional therapist, individuals can gain insight into their behaviors and patterns, develop coping skills, and cultivate resilience to navigate life's challenges more effectively. Therapy sessions may focus on addressing specific issues such as trauma recovery, anxiety management, depression treatment, relationship conflicts, or personal development goals. Therapists adapt their approach based on each client's unique strengths, preferences, and therapeutic needs. Regular therapy sessions provide ongoing support, encouragement, and guidance as individuals work toward healing, personal growth, and achieving their desired life goals.

Chapter Ten

Creating a Personal Somatic Therapy Plan

Creating a Personal Somatic Therapy Plan involves tailoring therapeutic practices to individual needs and goals, fostering healing, resilience, and personal growth through a holistic approach that integrates mind and body. This comprehensive plan encompasses assessing personal needs and goals, designing a customized practice routine, tracking progress, adjusting techniques as necessary, and overcoming challenges to maintain motivation and commitment to the therapeutic process.

Assessing Your Needs and Goals

Assessing Your Needs and Goals is the foundational step in creating a personal somatic therapy plan. It involves self-reflection, exploration of current challenges, and identification of desired outcomes for therapy. Individuals may assess various aspects of their lives, including emotional well-being, stress levels, physical health, relationship dynamics, and personal development goals.

Self-assessment involves identifying specific symptoms or issues that may benefit from somatic therapy, such as chronic stress, anxiety, trauma-related symptoms, or difficulties in emotional regulation. It also involves clarifying personal goals for therapy, such as improving overall well-being, enhancing resilience, developing coping skills, or healing from past experiences.

During this phase, individuals may benefit from consulting with a qualified somatic therapist or healthcare professional to gain insights into potential areas of focus and appropriate therapeutic approaches. Therapists can help individuals identify underlying patterns, triggers, and barriers to well-being, guiding them in formulating realistic and achievable goals for therapy.

Designing a Customized Practice Routine

Designing a Customized Practice Routine involves selecting and integrating somatic techniques that address identified needs and goals, creating a structured plan for regular practice and integration into daily life. A personalized routine typically includes a combination of somatic exercises, mindfulness practices, and self-care activities tailored to individual preferences, strengths, and therapeutic objectives. Somatic techniques may include body awareness exercises, breathwork, progressive muscle relaxation, somatic experiencing techniques, or mindful movement practices such as yoga or Tai Chi. These techniques help individuals cultivate greater awareness of bodily sensations, regulate physiological arousal, and promote relaxation and emotional healing.

Mindfulness practices complement somatic techniques by enhancing present-moment awareness, non-judgmental acceptance of thoughts and emotions, and compassionate self-awareness. Meditation practices such as body scan meditation, mindful breathing, or loving-kindness meditation support emotional regulation, stress reduction, and the integration of mind-body processes. Incorporating self-care activities into a personalized routine promotes holistic well-being and resilience. These activities may include adequate sleep, balanced nutrition, regular physical exercise, creative expression, social connection, and relaxation techniques such as journaling, spending time in nature, or engaging in hobbies that promote relaxation and enjoyment.

Tracking Progress and Adjusting Techniques

Tracking Progress and Adjusting Techniques involves monitoring therapeutic outcomes, evaluating the effectiveness of somatic practices, and making adjustments as needed to optimize healing and personal growth. Progress tracking allows individuals to reflect on their experiences, identify trends or changes in symptoms, and celebrate milestones achieved through somatic therapy. Individuals may use various methods to track progress, such as keeping a journal or diary to record thoughts, emotions, and physical sensations before and after somatic sessions. This practice helps individuals notice patterns, triggers, and improvements in well-being over time, providing valuable insights into the impact of somatic therapy on daily life.

Regular check-ins with a somatic therapist or healthcare provider support progress tracking by reviewing goals, discussing challenges or successes, and adjusting therapeutic strategies accordingly. Therapists may offer guidance on refining somatic techniques, exploring new approaches, or modifying practice routines to address evolving therapeutic needs and goals.

Adjusting techniques involves flexibility and openness to experimenting with different somatic practices or modifying existing routines based on individual preferences and responses. For example, individuals may explore variations of mindfulness meditation, try new somatic exercises, or incorporate additional self-care activities to enhance overall well-being and resilience.

Overcoming Challenges and Staying Motivated

Overcoming Challenges and Staying Motivated is essential for maintaining commitment to a personal somatic therapy plan over time. Challenges may arise during therapy, such as resistance to change, emotional discomfort, time constraints, or setbacks in progress. Developing resilience and coping strategies supports individuals in navigating challenges and sustaining motivation for therapeutic practice. Building a support network of friends, family members, or fellow therapy participants can provide encouragement, validation, and practical assistance during difficult times. Sharing experiences, seeking advice, and receiving empathy from others fosters a sense of connection and mutual support, enhancing motivation and resilience in the therapeutic journey.

Practicing self-compassion involves treating oneself with kindness, understanding, and acceptance during moments of struggle or self-doubt. Self-compassion cultivates emotional resilience, reduces self-criticism, and promotes a nurturing inner dialogue that supports perseverance and commitment to therapeutic goals. Setting realistic expectations for therapy involves acknowledging that healing and personal growth occur gradually and may involve periods of progress and setbacks. Embracing the process of change, learning from challenges, and celebrating small victories along the way promotes a positive outlook and sustained motivation for somatic therapy.

Exploring barriers to progress, such as fear of change, perfectionism, or self-limiting beliefs, allows individuals to develop strategies for overcoming obstacles and enhancing resilience. Therapists can offer guidance on addressing specific challenges, developing coping skills, and cultivating a growth mindset that supports resilience and adaptive coping strategies.

Chapter Eleven

Case Studies and Success Stories

Real-Life Examples of Somatic Healing

Real-Life Examples of Somatic Healing illustrate the transformative power of somatic therapy in addressing a wide range of psychological and physical challenges. These case studies highlight how somatic approaches, which integrate body-oriented techniques with psychological interventions, support individuals in healing from trauma, reducing stress, enhancing emotional regulation, and promoting overall well-being.

For instance, consider the case of Sarah, a survivor of childhood trauma who struggled with chronic anxiety and hypervigilance. Through somatic therapy sessions incorporating techniques such as Somatic Experiencing and mindfulness-based practices, Sarah learned to identify and release stored tension in her body associated with past traumatic experiences. Over time, Sarah reported a reduction in anxiety symptoms, improved sleep quality, and greater emotional resilience. By focusing on bodily sensations and regulating nervous system responses, somatic therapy helped Sarah reclaim a sense of safety and empowerment in her daily life.

Another example is James, who experienced chronic pain and emotional distress following a car accident. Traditional medical treatments provided limited relief, prompting James to explore somatic therapy as an alternative approach to pain management. Through sessions that included biofeedback, gentle movement exercises, and guided relaxation techniques, James learned to modulate his physical responses to pain and reduce emotional reactivity. As a result, James reported decreased pain intensity, improved mobility, and enhanced emotional well-being. Somatic therapy empowered James to cultivate self-care practices and regain a sense of control over his health and recovery journey.

These real-life examples demonstrate the holistic nature of somatic healing, emphasizing the interconnectedness of mind and body in promoting resilience and fostering personal growth. By addressing both physiological and psychological aspects of wellness, somatic therapy offers individuals like Sarah and James a pathway to healing, empowerment, and improved quality of life.

Interviews with Somatic Therapy Practitioners

Interviews with Somatic Therapy Practitioners provide valuable insights into the theoretical foundations, therapeutic techniques, and clinical applications of somatic approaches in mental health and wellness. Practitioners share their expertise, clinical experiences, and perspectives on the integration of body-oriented therapies with traditional psychotherapeutic modalities.

Dr. Maya Johnson, a licensed somatic therapist, discusses the principles of Somatic Experiencing and its application in trauma recovery. Dr. Johnson emphasizes the importance of tracking bodily sensations, facilitating nervous system regulation, and promoting safety and containment in therapeutic sessions. She explains how somatic techniques, such as pendulation and titration, help clients gradually process and integrate traumatic memories, supporting emotional healing and resilience.

In another interview, Dr. Michael Chen, a practitioner of Integrative Body-Mind Training (IBMT), explores the intersection of mindfulness meditation and somatic practices in promoting stress reduction and emotional well-being. Dr. Chen discusses IBMT's focus on cultivating mental clarity, enhancing self-regulation skills, and fostering mind-body integration through guided mindfulness practices and body-awareness techniques. He highlights research findings on IBMT's efficacy in improving attentional control, emotional regulation, and physiological health indicators.

These interviews with somatic therapy practitioners provide a nuanced understanding of how different approaches—such as Somatic Experiencing, Bioenergetic Analysis, and IBMT—address unique therapeutic goals and client populations. Practitioners share case examples, therapeutic insights, and ethical considerations in integrating somatic techniques with conventional psychotherapy, enhancing treatment outcomes and promoting holistic well-being.

Testimonials from Individuals Who've Benefited

Testimonials from Individuals Who've Benefited offer firsthand accounts of personal experiences with somatic therapy, highlighting the profound impact of these therapeutic approaches on emotional healing, personal growth, and resilience. Individuals share their journeys of overcoming challenges, discovering inner resources, and achieving transformative changes in their lives through somatic practices.

Emily, a survivor of domestic violence, shares how somatic therapy sessions helped her reconnect with her body and regain a sense of safety and empowerment. Through techniques such as grounding exercises and gentle movement, Emily learned to release physical tension and emotional distress associated with trauma.

She describes how somatic therapy enabled her to develop greater self-awareness, rebuild trust in her body, and cultivate healthier relationships.

John, a combat veteran suffering from post-traumatic stress disorder (PTSD), recounts his experience with somatic experiencing techniques. John explains how sessions focused on tracking bodily sensations and completing interrupted survival responses allowed him to gradually release stored trauma and reduce hyperarousal symptoms. He credits somatic therapy with helping him regain stability, improve sleep quality, and reconnect with his sense of purpose and resilience.

These testimonials underscore the transformative potential of somatic therapy in promoting recovery from trauma, managing stress-related symptoms, and enhancing overall well-being. Individuals express gratitude for the compassionate support, therapeutic guidance, and personalized care received from somatic therapists, highlighting the importance of a client-centered approach in fostering healing and empowerment.

By sharing their stories, individuals who have benefited from somatic therapy contribute to a growing narrative of resilience, hope, and personal empowerment. Their testimonials inspire others to explore somatic approaches, seek support for mental health challenges, and embrace holistic strategies for healing and well-being.

Conclusion

Congratulations on completing "Somatic Therapy Techniques for Beginners: The Proven Self-Soothing Handbook for Trauma Release, Mind-Body Balance, and Resilience Building." Throughout this journey, you've explored the transformative power of somatic practices—tools that empower you to navigate life's challenges with resilience, grace, and self-awareness. As you've learned, somatic therapy offers more than techniques; it's a philosophy rooted in the understanding that our bodies hold wisdom and healing potential. By tuning into physical sensations, regulating breath, and engaging in mindful movement, you've embarked on a path of profound self-discovery and growth.

Reflect on your experiences with grounding exercises, breathing techniques, and progressive muscle relaxation. Notice how these practices have supported you in releasing tension, calming your nervous system, and cultivating a deeper connection between mind and body. Each step you've taken has been a testament to your commitment to self-care and well-being. Remember, healing is not linear—it's a journey of peaks and valleys, moments of clarity and moments of challenge. As you continue to integrate somatic techniques into your daily life, be gentle with yourself. Embrace each moment as an opportunity for growth and learning, trusting in your innate capacity for resilience and transformation.

The stories of resilience and empowerment shared in this book serve as reminders that you are not alone on this path. Many have walked before you, overcoming obstacles, and finding strength in their journey toward healing. Let their experiences inspire you to persevere, to seek support when needed, and to honor your unique path to wellness. Whether you're navigating trauma recovery, seeking greater mind-body balance, or simply exploring new ways to enhance your well-being, know that somatic therapy offers a wealth of tools and insights to support you. Trust in the wisdom of your body, cultivate compassion for yourself, and celebrate each step forward on your journey.

Thank you for allowing "Somatic Therapy Techniques for Beginners" to be your companion in this transformative process. May you continue to nurture your mind-body connection, embrace your innate resilience, and live a life filled with vitality, authenticity, and profound self-discovery. Here's to your continued growth, healing, and well-being.

www.ingramcontent.com/pod-product-compliance
Lightning Source LLC
Chambersburg PA
CBHW071941210526
45479CB00002B/768